Living A Healthy

LIFESTYLE

BY

S.F OLA

ISBN-13:979-8-3752-4738-0

DEDICATION

" This book is dedicated to all those who are on a journey to improve their health and well-being. May it serve as a guide and inspiration for you to take control of your physical, mental, and emotional health, and to live a fulfilling and happy life. To all the warriors, who are fighting against the lifestyle-related health issues, may this book provide you with the knowledge and tools to take charge of your health and overcome the obstacles that come your way. To all of you who have the desire to improve your lifestyle and make it a habit, this book is for you. May it empower you to make informed choices and take positive steps towards a healthier, happier you."

Introduction:

In this book, we will explore the many different aspects of a healthy lifestyle and how to incorporate them into your daily routine. We will discuss the importance of exercise for overall health and well-being and provide tips for creating a healthy diet plan that includes whole foods, hydration, and portion control. We will also address common environmental and lifestyle-related health issues and how to manage them.

Additionally, we will delve into the importance of nutrition for overall health and well-being and discuss common mistakes to avoid when it comes to nutrition and how to overcome them. We will explore the negative impact of stress on overall health and well-being and provide tips for managing stress through mindfulness and relaxation techniques, time management, and setting boundaries. We will also discuss how to identify and address the root causes of stress.

We will also cover the importance of sleep and recovery for overall health and well-being and provide tips for improving sleep quality through creating a bedtime routine, avoiding screens before bed, and creating a comfortable sleep environment. We will also discuss how to incorporate rest and recovery into your daily routine.

We will also delve into the importance of mindfulness and mental health for overall health and well-being and provide tips for incorporating mindfulness practices into your daily routine, such as meditation, journaling, and yoga. We will also discuss how to address and manage common mental health issues.

We will also explore the impact of environment and lifestyle on overall health and well-being and discuss creating a healthy environment and how to address and manage common environmental and lifestyle-related health issues.

Finally, we will discuss the importance of prevention and self-care for overall health and well-being, and provide tips for incorporating preventative measures, such as regular check-ups and screenings, into your daily routine. We will also discuss how to practice self-care, such as setting boundaries, prioritizing self-care activities, and seeking support when needed.

By the end of this book, you will have a better understanding of how to live a healthy lifestyle and the tools you need to make positive changes in your life. We encourage you to act and start living a healthy lifestyle today.

TABLE OF CONTENTS   **Page**

CHAPTER ONE: HEALTHY LIFESTYLE AT A GLANCE

What a Healthy Lifestyle is and Why It is important

A healthy lifestyle is one that includes regular physical activity, a balanced diet, and adequate sleep. It also includes not smoking, limiting alcohol consumption, and managing stress. A healthy lifestyle is important because it can help reduce the risk of chronic diseases such as heart disease, diabetes, and cancer, as well as improve overall physical and mental well-being. Additionally, it can help improve quality of life, increase lifespan, and helps prevent chronic diseases. Therefore, it is important to make healthy choices to maintain a healthy lifestyle.

Overview of the different aspects of a healthy lifestyle

A healthy lifestyle encompasses many different aspects that work together to promote overall well-being. Here is an overview of some of the key areas:

- Exercise: Regular physical activity is important for maintaining good health. Exercise can help improve cardiovascular health, maintain a healthy weight, and reduce the risk of chronic diseases such as heart disease, diabetes, and cancer. Aim for at least 30 minutes of moderate-intensity physical activity, such as brisk walking, most days of the week.

- Nutrition: Eating a balanced diet that is rich in fruits, vegetables, whole grains, lean proteins, and healthy fats is important for providing the body with the nutrients and energy it needs. It's also important to limit the intake of added sugars, saturated and trans fats, and sodium.

- Sleep: Getting adequate sleep is important for overall health. Adults should aim for 7-9 hours of sleep per night. Lack of sleep can contribute to a variety of health problems, including obesity, diabetes, and heart disease.

- Stress management: Finding effective ways to manage stress can help prevent stress from becoming chronic and contributing to health problems. Techniques such as exercise, meditation, yoga, and therapy can help.

- Substance use: Limiting alcohol consumption and not smoking is important for maintaining a healthy lifestyle. Excessive alcohol consumption can lead to a variety of health problems, including liver disease, cancer, and mental health disorders. Smoking is one of the leading causes of preventable deaths worldwide.

- Mental and emotional well-being: A healthy lifestyle also includes activities that promote emotional well-being, such as maintaining relationships, participating in hobbies, and pursuing meaningful work.

- Preventive care: Regularly visiting healthcare professional for check-ups, screenings, and vaccinations, and taking steps to prevent illnesses, such as by practicing good hygiene, can help maintain good health.

It's important to note that maintaining a healthy lifestyle requires effort and commitment, but the benefits are well worth it. By making healthy choices and taking care of ourselves, we can reduce the risk of chronic diseases, improve our quality of life, and live longer, happier lives.

Setting healthy lifestyle goals and creating a plan to achieve them

It is important to set a realistic healthy lifestyle goal and creating a plan to achieve them in other to achieving and maintaining a healthy lifestyle. Here are some tips for setting and achieving healthy lifestyle goals:

1. Be specific: Clearly define what you want to achieve and set specific, measurable goals. For example, instead of saying "I want to eat healthier," set a goal to "eat at least five servings of fruits and vegetables per day."

2. Make them realistic: Your goals should be challenging but achievable. Avoid setting unrealistic goals that are unlikely to be met.

3. Set a timeline: Establish a deadline for achieving your goals. This will help you stay on track and make progress.

4. Create a plan: Once you have set your goals, create a plan that outlines the steps you will take to achieve them. Be sure to include specific actions, such as "I will go for a 30-minute walk every day at lunchtime."

5. Track your progress: Keep a record of your progress and adjust as needed. This will help you stay motivated and see how far you've come.

6. Get support: Surround yourself with people who will support and encourage you in your efforts to achieve your goals. Whether it's friends, family, or a health professional, having a support system can make a big difference.

7. Be flexible: Life happens, and sometimes goals change. Be open to adjusting your plan or your goals if necessary.

8. Reward yourself: Celebrate your successes along the way. Reward yourself when you achieve a goal or make progress towards one.

Remember, a healthy lifestyle is a journey, not a destination. So, be patient with yourself and don't get discouraged if you don't achieve your goals right away. The most important thing is to keep working towards them and make progress over time.

CHAPTER TWO: EXERCISE

Importance of exercise for overall health and well-being

Exercise is an important aspect of a healthy lifestyle and has many benefits for overall health and well-being.

- Physical health: Regular physical activity can help improve cardiovascular health, maintain a healthy weight, and reduce the risk of chronic diseases such as heart disease, diabetes, and cancer. Exercise can also improve muscle and bone strength, and increase flexibility and balance, which can reduce the risk of falls in older adults.

- Mental health: Exercise is also good for mental health. It can help reduce symptoms of depression and anxiety and improve mood. It can also reduce stress, improve cognitive function, and promote better sleep.

- Weight management: Regular exercise combined with a healthy diet can help you achieve and maintain a healthy weight. Physical activity can help burn calories and build muscle, which can increase metabolism.

- Quality of life: Regular exercise can help improve overall quality of life. It can improve energy levels, reduce fatigue, and improve overall fitness.

- Longevity: Exercise can also help increase lifespan, as it can reduce the risk of chronic diseases and improve overall health and well-being.

It's important to note that any type of physical activity can be beneficial and there is no need to start with intense workouts. You can start with a moderate-intensity physical activity such as brisk walking, cycling, swimming, dancing, or even house cleaning or gardening and gradually increasing the duration, frequency, and intensity of the activity over time. The important thing is to find an activity that you enjoy and stick with it.

Creating a healthy diet plan

Creating a healthy diet plan is an important step in maintaining a healthy lifestyle. Here are some tips for creating a healthy diet plan:

1. Focus on whole foods: Whole foods, such as fruits, vegetables, whole grains, lean proteins, and healthy fats, provide the nutrients and energy needed for good health. They are also less processed and contain fewer added sugars, saturated and trans fats, and sodium.

2. Hydration: Staying hydrated is important for overall health. Aim to drink at least 8-10 cups of water per day. You can also include other hydrating fluids such as herbal teas, coconut water, and low-fat milk.

3. Portion control: Eating the right amount of food is important for maintaining a healthy weight. Use smaller plates and be mindful of the amount of food you are consuming. You can also use measuring cups and food scales to ensure you are eating the correct portion sizes.

4. Plan your meals: Plan your meals and snacks in advance. This will help you stay on track and make healthy choices. Try to make meals at home as often as possible so you can control the ingredients and the portion sizes.

5. Limit processed foods: Processed foods are often high in added sugars, sodium, and unhealthy fats. Try to limit your intake of processed foods and opt for whole foods instead.

6. Include a variety of foods: Eating a variety of foods can help ensure you are getting all the necessary nutrients. Try to include a variety of fruits, vegetables, whole grains, lean proteins, and healthy fats in your diet.

7. Be mindful of calorie intake: Be aware of the total number of calories you are consuming each day. If you are trying to lose weight, you may need to consume fewer calories than you burn.

8. Consult with a professional: A dietitian or nutritionist can help you create a healthy diet plan that is tailored to your individual needs.

It's important to keep in mind that a healthy diet is not about strict restriction but about making healthy choices most of the time. A balanced diet allows for the occasional indulgence and should be enjoyable.

How to address and manage common environmental and lifestyle-related health issues

There are many environmental and lifestyle-related health issues that can negatively impact our well-being. Here are some tips for addressing and managing some common ones:

1. Air pollution: To reduce your exposure to air pollution, you can try to avoid heavy traffic, stay indoors on high pollution days, and use air purifiers in your home.

2. Noise pollution: To reduce your exposure to noise pollution, you can use earplugs or noise-canceling headphones, close windows, and doors to block out noise, and avoid loud environments.

3. Water pollution: To reduce your exposure to water pollution, you can filter your tap water, avoid swimming in potentially contaminated water, and be aware of local water quality reports.

4. Light pollution: To reduce your exposure to light pollution, you can use curtains or blinds to block out light, avoid looking at screens for several hours before bedtime, and use a sleep mask.

5. Sedentary lifestyle: To address the negative effects of a sedentary lifestyle, you can try to sit less and move more, take regular breaks to stand and walk around, and engage in regular physical activity.

6. Poor diet: To address the negative effects of a poor diet, you can try to eat a balanced diet that includes plenty of fruits, vegetables, whole grains, lean proteins, and healthy fats, and limit your intake of added sugars, saturated and trans fats, and sodium.

7. Stress: To address stress, you can try to practice stress-management techniques such as exercise, meditation, yoga, or therapy.

8. Substance use: To address substance use, you can try to reduce or quit smoking and drinking alcohol and seek professional help if needed.

It's important to note that addressing and managing environmental and lifestyle-related health issues may not always be easy, and it may require a combination of individual and community-level strategies. Consult with a health professional to determine the best course of action for addressing and managing your specific health concerns.

Incorporating exercise into your daily routine

Incorporating exercise into your daily routine can be challenging, but it is important for maintaining good health. Here are some tips for making exercise a regular part of your routine:

1. Make a schedule: Set aside specific times each day for exercise and make it a non-negotiable part of your daily routine.
2. Start small: Begin with a small amount of exercise and gradually increase the duration, frequency, and intensity over time.
3. Find an activity you enjoy: Choose an activity that you enjoy, whether it's walking, cycling, swimming, dancing, or even house cleaning or gardening.
4. Exercise with a friend: Find a workout partner to exercise with, it can be more fun, and you will be less likely to skip a workout.
5. Mix it up: Vary your workouts to keep it interesting. Try different types of exercise to avoid boredom.
6. Use technology: Use a fitness tracker or an app to track your progress, set goals, and stay motivated.
7. Get creative: Find ways to incorporate physical activity into your daily routine. For example, take the stairs instead of the elevator, walk or bike to work, or go for a walk during lunch breaks.

8. Be consistent: Make exercise a regular part of your routine. Even if you miss a day, don't give up, just get back on track the next day.

Remember, it can take time to develop an exercise routine, and everyone is different. But by starting small, finding an activity you enjoy, and being consistent, you'll be more likely to make exercise a regular part of your daily routine.

CHAPTER THREE: NUTRITION

Importance of nutrition for overall health and well-being

Nutrition plays a crucial role in overall health and well-being. A balanced diet, including the right balance of macronutrients (carbohydrates, proteins, and fats) and micronutrients (vitamins and minerals), is essential for maintaining good health and preventing chronic diseases.

- Physical health: A balanced diet can help maintain a healthy weight, provide the body with the energy it needs to function, and reduce the risk of chronic diseases such as heart disease, diabetes, and cancer. It also helps to prevent nutrient deficiencies, which can lead to a variety of health problems.

- Mental health: A good nutrition is also important for mental health. Eating a balanced diet can help improve mood and reduce symptoms of depression and anxiety.

- Cognitive function: Adequate intake of certain nutrients such as omega-3 fatty acids, vitamins B12 and D, and iron, can help to improve cognitive function and reduce the risk of cognitive decline.

- Bone health: A diet rich in calcium and vitamin D can help to maintain strong and healthy bones.

- Immune system: A healthy diet can help to support the immune system, which is important for fighting off infections and illnesses.

- Weight management: A healthy diet can help with weight management by providing the right balance of macronutrients and keeping you feeling full and satisfied.

It's important to note that a healthy diet is not only about the foods you eat but also about the way you eat. Eating mindfully and avoiding eating too quickly, eating until you are full, and eating at regular intervals are all important for overall health and well-being.

Creating a healthy diet plan

Creating a healthy diet plan is an important step in maintaining a healthy lifestyle. Here are some tips for creating a healthy diet plan:

1. Focus on whole foods: Whole foods, such as fruits, vegetables, whole grains, lean proteins, and healthy fats, provide the nutrients and energy needed for good health. They are also less processed and contain fewer added sugars, saturated and trans fats, and sodium.

2. Hydration: Staying hydrated is important for overall health. Aim to drink at least 8-10 cups of water per day. You can also include other hydrating fluids such as herbal teas, coconut water, and low-fat milk.

3. Portion control: Eating the right amount of food is important for maintaining a healthy weight. Use smaller plates and be mindful of the amount of food you are consuming. You can also use measuring cups and food scales to ensure you are eating the correct portion sizes.

4. Plan your meals: Plan your meals and snacks in advance. This will help you stay on track and make healthy choices. Try to make meals at home as often as possible so you can control the ingredients and the portion sizes.

5. Limit processed foods: Processed foods are often high in added sugars, sodium, and unhealthy fats. Try to limit your intake of processed foods and opt for whole foods instead.

6. Include a variety of foods: Eating a variety of foods can help ensure you are getting all the necessary nutrients. Try to include a variety of fruits, vegetables, whole grains, lean proteins, and healthy fats in your diet.

7. Be mindful of calorie intake: Be aware of the total number of calories you are consuming each day. If you are trying to lose weight, you may need to consume fewer calories than you burn.

8. Consult with a professional: A dietitian or nutritionist can help you create a healthy diet plan that is tailored to your individual needs.

9. Eat mindfully: Eating mindfully, paying attention to your hunger and fullness cues, and avoiding distractions while eating can help you make healthier food choices.

10. Experiment with different foods: Experiment with new foods, spices, and cooking methods to keep your meals interesting and enjoyable.

Remember, a healthy diet is not about strict restriction but about making healthy choices most of the time. A balanced diet allows for the occasional indulgence and should be enjoyable. Also, it's important to consider any allergies, intolerances or any medical condition that may affect your diet choices and consult with a professional if necessary.

Common mistakes to avoid when it comes to nutrition and how to overcome them

Making mistakes when it comes to nutrition is common, but they can be easily overcome with a little bit of knowledge and effort. Here are some common mistakes to avoid when it comes to nutrition and how to overcome them:

1. Skipping meals: Skipping meals can lead to overeating later and can disrupt your metabolism. To overcome this, try to eat regular meals and snacks at set times each day.

2. Restricting certain food groups: Restricting certain food groups, such as carbohydrates or fats, can lead to nutrient deficiencies and can be difficult to maintain over time. To overcome this, aim for a balanced diet that includes a variety of nutrient-dense foods.

3. Relying on processed foods: Processed foods are often high in added sugars, sodium, and unhealthy fats. To overcome this, try to limit your intake of processed foods and opt for whole foods instead.

4. Eating too much sugar: Consuming too much added sugar can lead to weight gain and an increased risk of chronic diseases. To overcome this, try to limit your intake of added sugars and opt for natural sweeteners like honey or maple syrup.

5. Not getting enough fiber: Not getting enough fiber can lead to constipation and an increased risk of chronic diseases. To overcome this, try to include more high-fiber foods in your diet, such as fruits, vegetables, whole grains, and legumes.

6. Not paying attention to portion sizes: Eating too much can lead to weight gain. To overcome this, use smaller plates, measure your food, and be mindful of the amount of food you are consuming.

7. Not reading labels: Not reading labels can lead to consuming too much sodium, sugar, and unhealthy fats. To overcome this, take the time to read labels and compare products to make healthier choices.

8. Not planning: This can lead to impulsive eating and poor food choices. To overcome this, plan your meals and snacks in advance, and have healthy options readily available.

Remember, a healthy diet is not about perfection, it's about progress. Making small changes and being consistent will help you to achieve your nutrition goals over time.

CHAPTER FOUR: STRESS MANAGEMENT

Negative impact of stress on overall health and well-being

Stress is a normal part of life, but when it becomes chronic, it can have a negative impact on overall health and well-being. Here are some ways that stress can affect your health:

1. Mental health: Chronic stress can lead to mental health problems such as anxiety and depression. It can also make existing mental health conditions worse.

2. Physical health: Stress can affect the body in many ways, including increasing the risk of heart disease, stroke, high blood pressure, and diabetes. Stress can also affect the immune system and make it harder for the body to fight off infections and illnesses.

3. Sleep: Stress can make it difficult to fall asleep and stay asleep, leading to insomnia and fatigue.

4. Digestive system: Stress can cause stomach upset and indigestion and can make conditions such as irritable bowel syndrome (IBS) and inflammatory bowel disease (IBD) worse.

5. Skin: Stress can cause acne and eczema flare-ups.

6. Reproductive system: Stress can affect the menstrual cycle and sexual function and can make it harder to conceive.

7. Cognitive function: Stress can affect cognitive function, including memory and concentration.

8. Weight: Stress can cause weight gain or weight loss and can make it harder to manage weight.

It's important to note that everyone experiences stress differently and the impact of stress on health can vary greatly from person to person. It's important to find ways to manage stress, such as exercise, meditation, yoga, therapy, or other stress-management techniques. If stress is affecting your daily life, it's important to seek help from a mental health professional.

Managing stress

Managing stress is important for overall health and well-being. Here are some tips for managing stress:

1. Mindfulness and relaxation techniques: Mindfulness practices such as meditation, yoga, and deep breathing can help to reduce stress and improve overall well-being. Relaxation techniques such as progressive muscle relaxation and guided imagery can also be helpful.

2. Time management: Prioritizing and managing time effectively can help to reduce stress caused by feeling overwhelmed. Try to break large tasks into smaller, manageable tasks and set realistic deadlines for yourself.

3. Setting boundaries: Setting boundaries can help to reduce stress caused by overcommitting and taking on too much. Learn to say no to non-essential tasks and activities and make time for self-care.

4. Exercise: Regular physical activity can help to reduce stress and improve overall well-being. Aim for at least 30 minutes of moderate-intensity exercise, such as brisk walking, cycling, or swimming, most days of the week.

5. Sleep: Getting enough sleep is important for managing stress. Aim for 7-9 hours of sleep per night and establish a regular sleep routine.

6. Eating well: Eating a healthy diet can help to reduce stress. Aim for a diet that includes plenty of fruits, vegetables, whole grains, lean proteins, and healthy fats.

7. Connecting with others: Connecting with others can help to reduce stress. Spend time with friends and family and consider joining a support group or participating in a social activity.

8. Seek professional help: If stress is affecting your daily life, consider seeking help from a mental health professional, such as a counselor, therapist, or psychiatrist.

Remember that stress is a normal part of life, and everyone's experience is unique. There's no one-size-fits-all solution, it's important to find what works for you, and be consistent with the techniques that help you to manage stress.

Identifying and addressing the root causes of stress

Stress can be caused by many different factors and identifying the root cause of stress is important for addressing it effectively. Here are some tips for identifying and addressing the root causes of stress:

1. Keep a stress journal: Record the situations or events that trigger stress, your physical and emotional reactions, and any coping strategies you used. This can help you identify patterns and potential root causes of stress.

2. Reflect on your thoughts and beliefs: Sometimes, stress can be caused by negative thoughts and beliefs. Reflect on your thoughts and beliefs and try to identify any that may be causing stress.

3. Evaluate your lifestyle: Stress can be caused by several lifestyle factors such as poor diet, lack of exercise, poor sleep, and substance use. Evaluate your lifestyle and make changes to improve your overall well-being.

4. Assess your relationships: Stress can be caused by relationship problems, whether it's with a significant other, family members, friends, or colleagues. Identify any relationships that may be causing stress and take steps to improve or end them if necessary.

5. Identify your values: Assess your values and priorities, and make sure that your actions align with them. When our actions don't align with our values and beliefs, it can lead to stress.

6. Seek professional help: If you are unable to identify the root cause of your stress or if you feel overwhelmed, consider seeking help from a mental health professional such as a counselor, therapist, or psychiatrist.

Once you have identified the root cause of stress, you can develop a plan to address it. This may include making lifestyle changes, seeking professional help, or learning stress-management techniques. It's important to be patient with yourself and to remember that change takes time.

CHAPTER FIVE: SLEEP AND RECOVERY

Importance of sleep and recovery for overall health and well-being

Sleep and recovery are essential for overall health and well-being. Here are some ways in which sleep, and recovery contribute to good health:

1. Physical health: Adequate sleep is essential for maintaining physical health. It helps to repair and rejuvenate the body, and it is essential for the immune system to function properly.

2. Mental health: Sleep is also essential for maintaining mental health. It helps to improve mood, reduce stress and anxiety, and improve cognitive function.

3. Athletic performance: Sleep is important for athletic performance. Adequate sleep helps to improve reaction time, endurance, and coordination.

4. Weight management: Sleep plays a role in weight management. Adequate sleep can help to regulate appetite and metabolism and may reduce the risk of obesity.

5. Safety: Lack of sleep can affect judgement and reaction time, increasing the risk of accidents and injuries.

6. Recovery: Sleep is essential for recovery after an illness or injury. During sleep, the body releases growth hormone which helps in the repair of damaged tissues and muscles.

7. Memory and learning: Adequate sleep is important for memory consolidation and learning. The brain processes and organizes new information learned during the day during sleep.

8. Sleep is also essential for the proper functioning of the cardiovascular, endocrine, and metabolic systems.

It's important to note that the quality of sleep is as important as the quantity. A regular sleep schedule, avoiding screens for 1 hour before bed, creating a comfortable sleep environment, and avoiding caffeine, nicotine and alcohol are some of the ways to improve the quality of sleep. Also, it's important to consult with a healthcare professional if you have trouble sleeping or staying asleep.

Tips for improving sleep quality

Improving sleep quality is essential for overall health and well-being. Here are some tips for improving sleep quality:

1. Create a bedtime routine: Having a consistent bedtime routine can help to signal to the body that it's time to sleep. This could include activities such as reading, listening to soothing music, or taking a warm bath.
2. Avoid screens before bed: The blue light emitted from screens can interfere with the production of melatonin, a hormone that regulates sleep. Try to avoid screens for at least an hour before bed.
3. Create a comfortable sleep environment: The environment in which you sleep can greatly affect the quality of your sleep. Keep the room dark, quiet, cool, and comfortable. Use a comfortable mattress and pillows.
4. Limit caffeine and alcohol: Caffeine and alcohol can affect the quality of sleep. Try to avoid consuming them in the hours leading up to bedtime.
5. Limit nicotine: Nicotine is a stimulant and can affect the quality of sleep.
6. Exercise regularly: Regular physical activity can help to improve sleep quality. However, it's important to avoid vigorous exercise close to bedtime.

7. Eat a healthy diet: Eating a healthy diet can help to improve sleep quality. Avoid eating large meals close to bedtime and try to avoid foods that can cause indigestion.

8. Relax before bed: Relaxation techniques such as deep breathing, progressive muscle relaxation, and yoga can help to reduce stress and prepare the body for sleep.

9. Establish a regular sleep schedule: Try to go to sleep and wake up at the same time every day, even on weekends, to help regulate the body's internal clock.

It's important to keep in mind that everyone is different, and it may take some time to find what works best for you. Also, it's important to consult with a healthcare professional if you have trouble sleeping or staying asleep.

How to incorporate rest and recovery into your daily routine

Incorporating rest and recovery into your daily routine is important for overall health and well-being. Here are some tips for incorporating rest and recovery into your daily routine:

1. Prioritize sleep: Make sure you are getting enough sleep each night. Aim for 7-9 hours of sleep per night and establish a regular sleep schedule.

2. Take breaks during the day: Taking short breaks during the day can help to reduce stress and improve productivity. Use this time to stretch, take a walk, or engage in a relaxing activity.

3. Schedule in relaxation time: Make time for relaxation and self-care activities such as reading, meditating, or taking a warm bath.

4. Practice mindfulness: Mindfulness practices such as meditation and yoga can help to reduce stress and improve overall well-being.

5. Listen to your body: Pay attention to your body's signals of fatigue and take a break when you need it.

6. Incorporate restorative exercise: Incorporate restorative exercise such as yoga, tai chi, or gentle stretching into your routine.

7. Get a massage: Massage therapy can help to reduce muscle tension and improve circulation.

8. Practice deep breathing: Deep breathing exercises can help to reduce stress and improve relaxation.

9. Make time for leisure activities: Engage in leisure activities that you enjoy such as hobbies, reading or listening to music.

10. Seek professional help: If you are having trouble incorporating rest and recovery into your daily routine, consider seeking help from a healthcare professional such as a counselor, therapist, or physician.

It's important to remember that rest and recovery are just as important as exercise and activity. Incorporating rest and recovery into your daily routine can help to improve overall health and well-being.

CHAPTER SIX: MINDFULNESS AND MENTAL HEALTH

Importance of mindfulness and mental health

Mindfulness and mental health are important for overall health and well-being. Here are some ways in which mindfulness and mental health contribute to good health:

1. Mental Health: Mindfulness practices such as meditation, yoga, and deep breathing can help to reduce stress, anxiety, and depression. These practices can also improve overall mental well-being and emotional regulation.

2. Physical health: Mindfulness practices have been shown to have a positive effect on physical health. They can lower blood pressure, improve immune function, and reduce pain.

3. Cognitive function: Mindfulness practices can improve cognitive function, including memory and attention.

4. Resilience: Mindfulness practices can help individuals to develop greater resilience in the face of stress and adversity.

5. Relationship: Mindfulness practices can improve communication and empathy, leading to better relationships.

6. Decision-making: Mindfulness practices can help individuals make better decisions by decreasing impulsiveness, increasing awareness of thoughts and emotions, and promoting rational thinking.

7. Self-awareness: Mindfulness practices can increase self-awareness, allowing individuals to gain insight into their thoughts, emotions, and behaviors.

8. Body awareness: Mindfulness practices can improve body awareness, allowing individuals to be more present in their bodies and to cultivate a deeper sense of well-being.

It's important to note that mindfulness practices are not a replacement for professional help, but they can be a helpful complement to therapy or medication. Mindfulness practices can be learned and practiced by anyone, and it's important to find the practices that work best for you and make them a regular part of your daily routine. There are many resources available to help you get started, such as guided meditations, mindfulness apps, and classes. It's also important to consult with a healthcare professional if you are experiencing severe mental health issues, such as depression or anxiety, or if you have a history of mental illness.

Incorporating mindfulness practices into your daily routine can help to improve overall health and well-being. It can also help to build a greater sense of self-awareness, which is essential for making positive changes in your life. Remember, like any skill, mindfulness takes practice, so be patient with yourself and give yourself time to adjust to the new routine.

Tips for incorporating mindfulness practices into your daily routine

Incorporating mindfulness practices into your daily routine can be a great way to improve overall health and well-being. Here are some tips for incorporating mindfulness practices into your daily routine:

1. Start small: Begin with just a few minutes of mindfulness practice each day and gradually increase the duration as you get more comfortable.

2. Make it a habit: Incorporate mindfulness practices into your daily routine, such as practicing meditation or yoga in the morning or journaling before bed.

3. Find what works for you: There are many different mindfulness practices, such as meditation, yoga, tai chi, and journaling. Experiment to find what works best for you.

4. Use guided meditations: Guided meditations can be helpful for beginners, as they provide structure and guidance. There are many free resources available online such as apps, videos, and audios.

5. Incorporate mindfulness into daily activities: Practice mindfulness during everyday activities such as cooking, eating, or taking a shower.

6. Create a designated space for practice: Create a designated space for your mindfulness practice, such as a corner of your room or a specific chair.

7. Get support: Consider joining a mindfulness class or finding a mindfulness partner to practice with.

8. Be consistent: Mindfulness practices require consistent practice to be most effective. Set aside some time each day to engage in mindfulness practices.

9. Be patient with yourself: Remember that developing mindfulness is a process and it takes time. Be patient and kind to yourself as you learn and grow.

10. Seek professional help: If you are experiencing severe mental health issues, such as depression or anxiety, or if you have a history of mental illness, it's important to seek professional help. Mindfulness practices can be a helpful complement to therapy or medication, but they are not a replacement for professional help. A mental health professional can provide guidance and support as you incorporate mindfulness practices into your daily routine.

It's important to remember that mindfulness practices are not a quick fix, but rather a lifelong journey. Incorporating mindfulness practices into your daily routine can help to improve overall health and well-being, but it takes time and consistent practice to see the benefits. Be patient with yourself and remember to be kind and compassionate towards yourself as you learn and grow.

How to address and manage common mental health issues

Mental health issues are common and can affect anyone. Here are some tips for addressing and managing common mental health issues:

1. Seek professional help: If you are experiencing severe mental health issues, such as depression or anxiety, it's important to seek professional help. A mental health professional can provide guidance, support, and treatment options.
2. Learn about your condition: Educating yourself about your condition can help you to better understand and manage it.
3. Create a self-care plan: Create a self-care plan that includes healthy habits such as exercise, healthy eating, and getting enough sleep.
4. Practice mindfulness: Mindfulness practices such as meditation, yoga, and deep breathing can help to reduce stress and improve overall well-being.
5. Connect with others: Connecting with others can help to reduce feelings of isolation and improve overall well-being.
6. Get support: Consider joining a support group or participating in a social activity.

7. Take medication as prescribed: If you are prescribed medication, take it as directed and follow up with your healthcare provider.

8. Limit alcohol and drug use: Alcohol and drug use can worsen mental health symptoms and should be avoided.

9. Take care of your physical health: Taking care of your physical health, through regular exercise and healthy eating, can have a positive impact on your mental health.

10. Be patient and kind to yourself: Remember that healing takes time and it's important to be patient and kind to yourself as you work towards recovery.

It's important to remember that everyone's experience with mental health issues is unique, and there is no one-size-fits-all solution. It's important to work with a mental health professional to develop an individualized plan that works best for you.

CHAPTER SEVEN: ENVIRONMENT AND LIFESTYLE

Impact of environment and lifestyle on overall health and well-being

The environment and lifestyle can have a significant impact on overall health and well-being. Here are some ways in which environment and lifestyle can affect health:

1. Air pollution: Exposure to air pollution can cause respiratory problems, heart disease, and cancer.

2. Water pollution: Exposure to contaminated water can cause a range of health problems, including gastrointestinal illness and reproductive problems.

3. Noise pollution: Exposure to loud noise can cause hearing loss, sleep disturbances, and cardiovascular disease.

4. Light pollution: Exposure to artificial light at night can disrupt the body's natural sleep-wake cycle and increase the risk of certain cancers and other health problems.

5. Environmental toxins: Exposure to environmental toxins such as lead, pesticides, and heavy metals can cause a range of health problems, including cancer and neurological damage.

6. Poor diet: A diet high in processed foods, sugar, and saturated fat can increase the risk of chronic diseases such as obesity, diabetes, and heart disease.

7. Lack of physical activity: A sedentary lifestyle can increase the risk of chronic diseases such as obesity, diabetes, and heart disease.

8. Smoking and alcohol consumption: Smoking and excessive alcohol consumption can increase the risk of cancer, heart disease, and liver disease.

9. Stress: Chronic stress can lead to a range of health problems, including heart disease, depression, and anxiety.

10. Lack of social support: Social isolation can lead to poor mental health and increase the risk of chronic diseases.

It's important to be aware of the impact of environment and lifestyle on overall health and to take steps to promote healthy living, such as eating a balanced diet, getting regular exercise, and avoiding harmful substances. Additionally, it's important to advocate for policies that promote a healthy environment and to support organizations that work to protect public health.

Creating a healthy environment

Creating a healthy environment is important for overall health and well-being. Here are some ways to create a healthy environment:

1. Improve indoor air quality: Use natural cleaning products, keep the humidity level low, and use plants to purify the air.

2. Reduce exposure to toxins: Avoid using products that contain harmful chemicals such as pesticides, lead, and heavy metals.

3. Improve water quality: Use a water filter and test your water for contaminants.

4. Promote natural light: Maximize the use of natural light in your home or workplace by keeping windows clean and removing heavy curtains or blinds.

5. Minimize noise pollution: Use earplugs or noise-cancelling headphones and try to avoid loud noises as much as possible.

6. Encourage physical activity: Create a space for physical activity in your home or workplace, such as a home gym or a designated walking area.

7. Promote healthy eating: Create a space for growing your own fruits and vegetables or invest in a water filter to ensure that the water you drink is clean and healthy.

8. Promote social connections: Encourage social connections by creating spaces for socializing in your home or workplace.

9. Promote mental well-being: Create a calm and relaxing environment by using soothing colors and textures and incorporating natural elements such as plants.

10. Encourage sustainable living: Encourage sustainable living by investing in energy-efficient appliances and recycling.

It's important to note that creating a healthy environment is an ongoing process and requires regular attention and maintenance. It's also important to keep in mind that everyone's needs, and preferences are different, so it's important to find what works best for you.

How to address and manage common environmental and lifestyle-related health issues

Common environmental and lifestyle-related health issues can have a significant impact on overall health and well-being. Here are some ways to address and manage these issues:

1. Air pollution: Limit exposure to air pollution by staying indoors on days when the air quality is poor and by avoiding areas with heavy traffic. Use air purifiers in your home and workplace.

2. Water pollution: Use a water filter to ensure that the water you drink is clean and healthy. Avoid swimming in water that may be contaminated.

3. Noise pollution: Limit exposure to loud noise by using earplugs or noise-cancelling headphones and try to avoid loud noises as much as possible.

4. Light pollution: Use curtains or blinds to block out artificial light at night and encourage the use of natural light during the day.

5. Environmental toxins: Use natural cleaning products and avoid using products that contain harmful chemicals such as pesticides, lead, and heavy metals.

6. Poor diet: Adopt a healthy diet that includes whole foods, fruits, vegetables, lean proteins, and healthy fats.

7. Lack of physical activity: Engage in regular physical activity and try to incorporate movement into your daily routine.

8. Smoking and alcohol consumption: Avoid smoking and limit alcohol consumption to reduce the risk of chronic diseases.

9. Stress: Practice stress management techniques such as mindfulness, exercise, and relaxation.

10. Lack of social support: Build and maintain strong social connections through activities, hobbies, and relationships.

It's important to note that addressing and managing environmental and lifestyle-related health issues requires a comprehensive approach and a commitment to making positive changes. It's also important to consult with a healthcare professional if you are experiencing severe health issues or if you have a history of chronic diseases.

CHAPTER EIGHT: PREVENTION AND SELF CARE

Importance of prevention and self-care for overall health and well-being

Prevention and self-care are important for overall health and well-being. Here are some ways in which prevention and self-care can contribute to good health:

1. Early detection: Regular check-ups, screenings, and tests can help to detect potential health issues early, which can make treatment more effective.

2. Health promotion: Adopting healthy habits such as eating a balanced diet, getting regular exercise, and avoiding harmful substances can help to promote overall health and well-being.

3. Stress management: Engaging in stress management techniques such as mindfulness, exercise, and relaxation can help to reduce stress and improve overall well-being.

4. Self-awareness: Self-awareness allows individuals to gain insight into their thoughts, emotions, and behaviors, which can help to identify and address potential health issues.

5. Empowerment: Self-care and prevention promote a sense of empowerment and control over one's health, which can lead to greater motivation to make positive changes.

6. Disease prevention: Adopting healthy habits can help prevent chronic diseases such as heart disease, diabetes, and cancer.

7. Mental health promotion: Self-care practices such as mindfulness and social connections can help to promote mental well-being.

8. Cost-effective: Preventive care can often be more cost-effective than treatment of an existing health issue.

9. Quality of life: A good health is essential for a good quality of life, and self-care and prevention can help to improve overall health and well-being.

10. Lifelong approach: Prevention and self-care are a lifelong approach to health and well-being, and the benefits are cumulative.

It's important to remember that prevention and self-care require a commitment to making positive changes and to maintaining healthy habits over time. It's also important to consult with a healthcare professional to develop an individualized plan that considers any unique health concerns.

Tips for incorporating preventative measures

Incorporating preventative measures, such as regular check-ups and screenings, into your daily routine is an important aspect of maintaining overall health and well-being. Here are some tips for incorporating preventative measures into your daily routine:

1. Schedule regular check-ups: Schedule regular check-ups with your primary care physician and dentist and keep track of any recommended screenings or tests that are specific to your age and health history.

2. Keep track of your health: Keep track of your health by monitoring symptoms, changes in your body and maintaining a journal of your health.

3. Be proactive: Be proactive about your health by taking preventative measures such as getting enough sleep, eating a balanced diet and exercise.

4. Keep your immunizations up to date: Keep your immunizations up to date, as some of them are only recommended every couple of years.

5. Use preventive services: Take advantage of preventive services such as cancer screenings, and other preventive screenings when appropriate.

6. Make use of technology: Use technology to help you keep track of your health, such as apps that track your symptoms, remind you of appointments, and provide information about your condition.

7. Listen to your body: Listen to your body and pay attention to any changes or symptoms. If you experience any unusual symptoms, it's important to consult with a healthcare professional.

8. Self-examination: Learn how to do self-examination, such as breast or testicular self-examination, and do them regularly.

9. Be informed: Be informed about your health and the health of your family, by learning about the conditions that run in your family and the preventive measures that can be taken to reduce the risk.

10. Seek professional help: If you are experiencing severe health issues, it's important to seek professional help, and to consult with a healthcare professional to develop an individualized plan that takes into account any unique health concerns.

It's important to remember that prevention is a lifelong approach to health and well-being, and the benefits are cumulative. Consult with a healthcare professional to develop an individualized plan that works best for you.

How to practice self-care

Practicing self-care is an important aspect of maintaining overall health and well-being. Here are some tips for practicing self-care:

1. Set boundaries: Learn to set boundaries with others and say "no" when necessary. This can help to reduce stress and prevent burnout.

2. Prioritize self-care activities: Make time for self-care activities such as exercise, mindfulness, and hobbies. Schedule them into your daily routine and make them a priority.

3. Create a self-care plan: Create a self-care plan that includes healthy habits such as exercise, healthy eating, and getting enough sleep.

4. Take time for yourself: Take time for yourself, whether it's taking a relaxing bath, reading a book, or going for a walk.

5. Seek support: Don't hesitate to seek support from friends, family, or a healthcare professional if you need it.

6. Identify triggers: Identify triggers that cause stress or negative emotions and try to avoid or manage them.

7. Be kind to yourself: Be kind and compassionate towards yourself. Avoid self-criticism and try to focus on self-acceptance.

8. Find balance: Find balance in your life by creating a balance between your responsibilities, social life, and your personal needs.

9. Get enough sleep: Get enough sleep to help improve your overall well-being and to help you feel refreshed and energized.

10. Make self-care a priority: Make self-care a priority by setting realistic goals and taking small steps towards them. Remember that progress is progress, no matter how small.

It's important to remember that self-care is an ongoing process, and it's important to be patient with yourself and to make it a consistent part of your daily routine. It's also important to remember that self-care looks different for everyone, so it's important to find what works best for you. Finally, it's important to seek professional help if you are struggling with mental health issues or if you have a history of chronic diseases. A healthcare professional can provide guidance and support as you incorporate self-care practices into your daily routine.

CHAPTER NINE: CONCLUSION

A summary of the main points covered in the book

Overall, maintaining a healthy lifestyle is essential for overall health and well-being. This includes regular exercise, which can improve cardiovascular health, strengthen muscles and bones, and reduce stress. It also includes a healthy diet, which should include whole foods, adequate hydration, and appropriate portion sizes. Additionally, it's important to address and manage environmental and lifestyle-related health issues, such as air and water pollution, noise pollution, and exposure to toxins. Mindfulness and mental health are also important for overall health and well-being, and can be promoted through practices such as meditation, yoga, and journaling. Sleep and recovery are also crucial for overall health and well-being and can be promoted through good sleep hygiene and regular rest and recovery. Incorporating preventative measures, such as regular check-ups and screenings, into your daily routine is also important for maintaining overall health and well-being. Finally, practicing self-care, such as setting boundaries, prioritizing self-care activities, and seeking support when needed, can also contribute to overall health and well-being. It's also important to create a healthy environment that includes improving indoor air quality, reducing exposure to toxins, promoting natural light, minimizing noise pollution, and encouraging sustainable living.

Courage to act and start living a healthy lifestyle today

It's never too late to start living a healthy lifestyle. The benefits of regular exercise, healthy eating, and stress management are well-documented and can have a positive impact on your overall health and well-being. By taking small steps towards a healthier lifestyle, you can make a big difference in the long run. Start by setting realistic goals and deciding to achieve them. Incorporating physical activity into your daily routine, whether it's a brisk walk or a gym session, can help to improve cardiovascular health, strengthen muscles and bones, and reduce stress. Eating a balanced diet that includes whole foods, fruits, vegetables, lean proteins, and healthy fats can help to promote overall health and well-being. Addressing and managing environmental and lifestyle-related health issues, such as air and water pollution, noise pollution, and exposure to toxins, can also have a positive impact on your overall health and well-being. Don't be afraid to seek professional help if you are struggling with mental health issues or if you have a history of chronic diseases. Remember that a healthy lifestyle is a lifelong approach to health and well-being and it's worth it to start today.

Glossaries

Below is a list of terms and definitions that are used in this book, along with a brief explanation of their meaning:

- Exercise: Physical activity that is done with the goal of becoming stronger, healthier, and more fit. Examples include running, swimming, weightlifting, and cycling.
- Nutrition: The study of how food and drink affect the body, including how the body uses nutrients and how different nutrients interact with one another.
- Stress Management: Techniques used to manage and cope with stress, such as mindfulness, relaxation techniques, time management, and setting boundaries.
- Mindfulness: The practice of being present and fully engaged in the current moment, without judgment.
- Mental Health: The overall well-being of an individual's mind and emotions, including the ability to cope with stress, to form and maintain relationships, and to function in daily life.
- Self-care: The act of taking care of oneself, including physical, mental, and emotional well-being.
- Preventative Measures: actions taken to prevent illness or injury, such as regular check-ups and screenings.
- Sleep: A state of rest for the body and mind, during which the body repairs itself and the mind processes information.
- Recovery: The process of repairing and rebuilding the body after exercise or other physical activity.
- Hydration: The process of replenishing the body's fluids, which are essential for maintaining proper bodily function.

- Whole foods: Foods that are minimally processed and are as close to their natural state as possible.

- Portion Control: The practice of eating the appropriate amount of food for one's needs and goals.

- Environmental Health: The study of how the environment impacts human health and well-being.

- Lifestyle-related health issues: health problems that are caused by or are made worse by a person's lifestyle, such as poor diet, lack of physical activity, and smoking.

- Root Causes: the underlying cause or causes of a particular problem or issue.

- Mindfulness practices: Techniques used to cultivate mindfulness, such as meditation, journaling, and yoga.